Supernatural Beauty Prayer

God's Promises for Beauty & Grooming

Dy Wakefield

Cover Image: Image by Andreas Lischka from Pixabay

ISBN: 9798370079597

Thanks and Honor

To God Be the Glory (God, Jesus & the Holy Ghost)

****

Abba Father, I dedicate this book to You. I honor you with this book and all its portions. May this book which is referencing Your Word (Bible) do according to Psalm 107:20 KJV, "He sent his word, and healed them, and delivered them from their destructions." May this book and its anointing transform the lives, the bodies, the minds, the emotions of the readers who will in turn give You Glory. As the Holy Ghost quicken their mortal bodies (Romans 8:11) in Jesus Name.

****

Psalm 27:4 NIV To gaze upon the beauty of the LORD.

Isaiah 33:17 KJV Your eyes will see the king in his beauty.

~ For I will restore health to you And heal you of your wounds,' says the LORD, 'Because they called you an outcast saying: "This is Zion; No one seeks her." Jeremiah 30:17 NKJV

Contents

Intro

This book consists of a Supernatural Beauty Prayer plus a breakdown of all God's promises on different areas pertaining to Beauty & Grooming, Intimacy issues for Married Couples and so much more.

Read the prayer aloud and once you finish agree with it by saying, "I believe I receive it, Amen."

Go to the section pertaining to YOU and find things you would like healed or restored in your body, even some things you would never think God would care about. There are things you may not feel uncomfortable talking to others about but God knows you desire it. It may seem embarrassing to you but God can bring wholeness to you in those areas. Look at a condition you have and see the scripture that will supernaturally heal, restore and make you whole.

Take the word of God His promises on any area related to your need, want and desire and read it daily even put your name in to make it your own so it can become real to you. You can also record it and listen to it often. You have to allow the Word of God to consume you so when you wake up you see it, when you sleep you dream about, or just going about your day you can see what you are believing for as reality but it hasn't manifested yes. Hebrews 11:1 Now faith is the substance of things hoped for, the evidence of things not seen.

Just remain in faith "belief" and watch God transform your life and body. He said, "I'll stick with you until I've done everything I promised you," (Genesis 28:15 MSG).

I will give thanks to You, because I am awesomely and wonderfully made; Wonderful are Your works, And my soul knows it very well.
Psalm 139:14 NASB

Female "Beauty"

You are altogether beautiful, my darling.
Song of Solomon 4:7 NIV

To give them Beauty for Ashes. Isaiah 61:3 NKJV

Please note some of these scriptures may have different meanings but I am using what is stated by the scripture version given.

<u>FACE</u>

Song of Songs 1:15 NIV How beautiful you are, my darling! Oh, how beautiful!

Esther 2:7 CSB The young woman (Esther) was extremely good-looking.

Esther 2:7 NIV This young woman, who was also known as Esther, was beautiful.

Beautiful Complexion
Song of Solomon 4:7 AMP There is no flaw nor blemish in you!

Beautiful Eyes
Song of Solomon 7:4 NLT Your eyes are like the sparkling pools in Heshbon by the gate of Bath-rabbim.

Perfect Nose
Song of Solomon 7:4 NLT Your nose is as fine as the tower of Lebanon overlooking Damascus.

Beautiful Smile
Song of Solomon 4:3 NIV Your mouth is lovely.

Full Set of Teeth
Song of Solomon 4:2 CEV Your teeth…they match perfectly, not one is missing.

<u>HAIR</u>

God knows Your Hair is Important to You
Luke 12:7 KJV Indeed, the very hairs of your head are all numbered. Don't be afraid; you are worth more than many sparrows.

Matthew 10:30 KJV And even the very hairs of your head are all numbered.

Instant Hair Growth
Judges 16:22 GNT But his hair started growing back.

Hair loss
Luke 21:18 KJV But not a hair of your head will perish.

Benefits of Protein for Your Hair
Acts 27:34 KJV Wherefore I pray you to take some meat: for this is for your health: for there shall not an hair fall from the head of any of you. {Protein helps your hair grow and strengthen it}.

Long Hair

Song of Solomon 4:1, 6:5 NKJV Your hair is like a flock of goats, Going down from Mount Gilead.

1 Corinthians 11:15 NKJV But if a woman has long hair, it is a glory to her; for her hair is given to her for a covering.

Song of Solomon 7:5 NLT The sheen of your hair radiates royalty. The king is held captive by its tresses.

Healthy Hair

Song of Solomon 7:5 NLT Your head is as majestic as Mount Carmel, and the sheen of your hair radiates royalty. The king is held captive by its tresses.

BODY

Youthful Neck

Song of Solomon 4:4 NIV Your neck is like the tower of David.

Song of Solomon 7:4 NLT Your neck is as beautiful as an ivory tower.

Perky Breasts

Song of Solomon 4:5 NIV Your breasts are like two fawns, like twin fawns of a gazelle that browse among the lilies.

Song of Solomon 7:7 NLT Your breasts are like its clusters of fruit.

Perfect Navel

Song of Solomon 7:2 NLT Your navel is perfectly formed like a goblet filled with mixed wine.

Shapely Thighs

Song of Solomon 7:1 NLT O queenly maiden. Your rounded thighs are like jewels, the work of a skilled craftsman.

Curvy Hips

Song of Solomon 7:1 AMP The curves of your hips are like jewels, The work of the hands of an artist.

Healthy Shape (Weight)

Song of Solomon 7:7 NLT You are slender like a palm tree.

Esther 2:7 CSB The young woman had a beautiful figure.

Esther 2:7 NIV This young woman, who was also known as Esther, had a lovely figure.

<u>SKIN</u>

Skin Restoration
Job 33:25 NIV Let their flesh be renewed like a child's; let them be restored as in the days of their youth.

2 King 5:14 KJV and his flesh were restored like the flesh of a little child and he was clean

2 Samuel 14:25 NIV from the top of his head to the soles of his feet there was no blemish in him

Age Reversal
Psalm 103:5 NKJV Who satisfies your mouth with good things, So that your youth is renewed like the eagle's.

Beauty Treatments
Esther 2:3 NIV Let beauty treatments be given to them.

Esther 2:12 NIV She had to complete twelve months of beauty treatments prescribed for the women, six months with oil of myrrh.

Soft Skin
Song of Solomon 7:2 MSG Your skin is silken and tawny like a field of wheat touched by the breeze.

COSMETICS

Eye Makeup
Song of Solomon 4:1 NIV Your eyes behind your veil are doves.

Lipstick
Song of Solomon 4:3 NIV Your lips are like a scarlet ribbon.

Cosmetics
Esther 2:12 NIV She had to complete twelve months of beauty treatments prescribed for the women, six months with oil of myrrh and six with perfumes and cosmetics.

FRAGRANCE

Song of Solomon 4:10 NIV Fragrance of your perfume

Song of Solomon 4:11 NKJV And the fragrance of your garments Is like the fragrance of Lebanon.

Esther 2:12 NLT She was given the prescribed twelve months of beauty treatments—six months with oil of myrrh, followed by six months with special perfumes and ointments.

<u>BEAUTY TREATMENTS</u>

Apothecary Therapy

Jeremiah 8:22 KJV Is there no balm in Gilead?

Song of Solomon 4:13-14 KJV Thy plants are an orchard of pomegranates, with pleasant fruits; camphire, with spikenard, Spikenard and saffron; calamus and cinnamon, with all trees of frankincense; myrrh and aloes, with all the chief spices.

Genesis 37:25 NIV As they sat down to eat their meal, they looked up and saw a caravan of Ishmaelites□comingfrom Gilead.□Theircamels were loaded with spices, balm□, and myrrh,□andthey were on their way to take them down to Egypt.

Jeremiah 46:11 NIV Go up to Gilead and get balm

Light Therapy

For Skin, Eyes, Teeth

Hebrews 1:3 AMPC He is the sole expression of the glory of God [the Light-being, the out-raying or radiance of the divine].

Water Therapy

Internal

John 7:38 KJV He that believeth on me, as the scripture hath said, out of his belly shall flow rivers of living water.

Water Therapy

External

2 King 5:14 NLT So Naaman went down to the Jordan River and dipped himself seven times, as the man of God had instructed him. And his skin became as healthy as the skin of a young child, and he was healed!

Vaginal Therapy

Song of Solomon 4:12 NIV You are a garden locked up, my sister, my bride; you are a spring enclosed, a sealed fountain.

Body scrubs Dead Sea salt

Ezekiel 47:8-11 NIV [8]said to me, "This water flows toward the eastern region and goes down into the Arabah, where it enters the Dead Sea. When it empties into the sea, the salty water there becomes fresh. [9]Swarms of living creatures will live wherever the river flows. There will be large numbers of fish, because this water flows there and makes the salt water fresh; so where the river flows everything will live. [10]Fishermen will stand along the shore; from En Gedi to En Eglaim there will be places for spreading nets. The fish will be of many kinds—like the fish of the Mediterranean Sea. [11]But the swamps and marshes will not become fresh; they will be left for salt.

<u>HYGIENE</u>

Bathing

Proverbs 30:12 MSG Don't imagine yourself to be quite presentable when you haven't had a bath in weeks

Teeth

For White Teeth

Song of Solomon 4:2 CEV Your teeth are whiter than sheep freshly washed.

Breath

Song of Solomon 7:8 MSG Your breath is clean and cool like fresh mint

Hands

Song of Solomon 5:5 NI. My hands dripped with myrrh

Feet

Song of Solomon 7:1 NIV How beautiful your sandaled feet.

Song of Solomon 5:3 NASB I have washed my feet, How can I dirty them again?

GENITALS

Song of Solomon 4:13-14 NLT [13]Your thighs shelter a paradise of pomegranates with rare spices— henna with nard, [14]nard and saffron, fragrant calamus and cinnamon, with all the trees of frankincense, myrrh, and aloes, and every other lovely spice.

Song of Solomon 7:2 NLT Between your thighs lies a mound of wheat bordered with lilies.

FASHION & ACCESSORIES

Clothings enhances your beauty, it gives you confidence even when wearing the right bra.

Apparel

Esther 5:1 KJV Now it came to pass on the third day, that Esther put on [her] royal [apparel].

Luke 7:25 NIV Those who wear expensive clothes and indulge in luxury are in palaces.

Proverbs 31:22 KJV Her clothing is silk and purple.

Ezekiel 16:13 NLT Your clothes were made of fine linen and costly fabric and were beautifully embroidered.

Psalm 45:13 BST All her glory is that of the daughter of the king of Esebon, robed as she is in golden fringed garments.

Jewelry

Song of Songs 1:10 NIV Your cheeks are beautiful with earrings, your neck with strings of jewels..

Jewelry (continued)

Song of Solomon 4:4 NIV Your neck is like the tower of David, built with courses of stone; on it hang a thousand shields, all of them shields of warriors.

Song of Solomon 4:9 NIV Jewel of your necklace.

Esther 2:17 NLT And the king loved Esther more than any of the other young women. He was so delighted with her that he set the royal crown on her head and declared her queen instead of Vashti.

Genesis 24:22 NLT He took out a gold ring for her nose and two large gold bracelets for her wrists.

Ezekiel 16:13 NLT And so you were adorned with gold and silver.

Ezekiel 16:12 KJV And I put a jewel on thy forehead, and earrings in thine ears, and a beautiful crown upon thine head.

Psalm 45:9 NLT Kings' daughters are among your noble women. At your right side stands the queen, wearing jewelry of finest gold from Ophir!

Male "Handsome"

Please note some of these scriptures may have different meanings but I am using what is stated by the scripture version given.

<u>FACE</u>

Psalm 45:2 NLT You are the most handsome of all. Gracious words stream from your lips. God himself has blessed you forever.

Healthy Skin
2 Samuel 14:25 NKJV From the sole of his foot to the crown of his head there was no blemish in him.

Song of Solomon 5:13 MSG His face is rugged.

Song of Solomon 5:13 WYC His face is smooth and bronzed

Sexy Eyes
Song of Solomon 5:12 CEV His eyes are a pair of doves bathing in a stream flowing with milk.

Sexy Smile
Song of Solomon 5:16 KJV His mouth is most sweet.

Full Set of Teeth
Song of Solomon 4:2 CEV Your teeth…they match perfectly, not one is missing.

HAIR

God knows Your Hair is Important to You
Luke 12:7 Indeed, the very hairs of your head are all numbered. Don't be afraid; you are worth more than many sparrows.

Matthew 10:30 And even the very hairs of your head are all numbered.

Instant Hair Growth
Judges 16:22 GNT But his hair started growing back.

Hair Loss
Luke 21:18 But not a hair of your head will perish.

Benefits of Protein for Your Hair
Acts 27:34 KJV Wherefore I pray you to take some meat: for this is for your health: for there shall not an hair fall from the head of any of you. {Protein helps your hair grow and strengthen it}

Long hair

Judges 13:5 CSB For indeed, you will conceive and give birth to a son. You must never cut his hair, because the boy will be a Nazirite to God from birth, and he will begin to save Israel from the power of the Philistines.

2 Samuel 14:26 GNT His hair was very thick, and he had to cut it once a year, when it grew too long and heavy. It would weigh about five pounds according to the royal standard of weights.

2 Samuel 14:26 ERV At the end of every year, Absalom cut the hair from his head and weighed it. The hair weighed about five pounds.

Song of Solomon 5:11 MSG With raven black curls tumbling across his shoulders.

Song of Solomon 5:11 YLT His locks flowing, dark as a raven,

<u>BODY</u>

Strong Arms

Song of Solomon 5:14 ERV His arms are like gold rods

Nice Hands

Song of Solomon 5:14 GNT His hands are well-formed

Six Pack

Song of Solomon 5:14 AMP His abdomen is a figure of carved ivory Inlaid with sapphires.

Song of Solomon 5:14 MSG His torso is the work of a sculptor, hard and smooth as ivory.

Big Chest

Song of Solomon 5:14 GW His chest is a block of ivory covered with sapphires.

Good Posture

Song of Solomon 5:15 MSG He stands tall, like a cedar, strong and deep-rooted

Strong Legs

Song of Solomon 5:15 KJV His legs are as pillars of marble, set upon sockets of fine gold:

Healthy Physique (Weight)

Song of Solomon 2:9 AMP My beloved is like a gazelle or a young stag.

Song of Solomon 5:10 MSG My dear lover glows with health— red-blooded, radiant!

Song of Solomon 5:10 HCSB My love is fit and strong.

Song of Solomon 5:10 CEV He is handsome and healthy.

Song of Solomon 5:14 MSG Fine muscles ripple beneath his skin, quiet and beautiful.

Song of Solomon 5:14 VOICE His body displays his manhood like an ivory tusk inlaid with sapphires.

<u>SKIN</u>

Skin Restoration
Job 33:25 NLT Then his body will become as healthy as a child's, firm and youthful again.

2 King 5:14 KJV And his flesh were restored like the flesh of a little child and he was clean

2 Samuel 14:25 NIV From the top of his head to the soles of his feet there was no blemish in him

Age Reversal

Psalm 103:5 NKJV Who satisfies your mouth with good things, So that your youth is renewed like the eagle's.

FRAGRANCE

Song of Solomon 1:3 NET The fragrance of your colognes is delightful.

Song of Solomon 5:15 MSG A rugged mountain of a man, aromatic with wood and stone.

Psalm 45:8 KJV All thy garments smell of myrrh, and aloes, and cassia

HYGIENE

Bathing

Proverbs 30:12 MSG Don't imagine yourself to be quite presentable when you haven't had a bath in weeks.

Body

Song of Solomon 1:3 NIRV The lotion you have on pleases me.

Teeth

White Teeth

Song of Solomon 4:2 CEV Your teeth are whiter than sheep freshly washed.

Breath

Song of Solomon 5:13 VOICE His lips are lilies dripping and flowing with myrrh.

Song of Solomon 7:8 MSG Your breath is clean and cool like fresh mint.

Hair

Song of Solomon 5:2 GNT My head is wet with dew, and my hair is damp from the mist.

Beard

Song of Solomon 5:13 MSG His beard smells like sage.

Song of Solomon 5:13 VOICE His bearded cheeks are like a spice garden, with towers of spice

Feet

Romans 10:15 KJV As it is written, How beautiful are the feet of them that preach the gospel of peace, and bring glad tidings of good things!

FASHION & ACCESSORIES

Apparel

Esther 6:8 KJV Let the royal apparel be brought which the king [useth] to wear.

Acts 12:21 KJV And upon a set day Herod, arrayed in royal apparel.

Luke 7:25 NIV Those who wear expensive clothes and indulge in luxury are in palaces.

Exodus 39:1 NLT The craftsmen made beautiful sacred garments of blue, purple, and scarlet cloth—clothing for Aaron to wear while ministering in the Holy Place, just as the LORD had commanded Moses.

Exodus 39:27-28 NLT [27]They made tunics for Aaron and his sons from fine linen cloth. [28]The turban and the special head coverings were made of fine linen, and the undergarments were also made of finely woven linen.

Genesis 41:42 NIV Then Pharaoh dressed (Joseph) in robes of fine linen.

Luke 15:22 NIV But the father said to his servants, 'Quick! Bring the best robe and put it on him…and sandals on his feet.

Daniel 5:29 NLT Then at Belshazzar's command, Daniel was dressed in purple robes.

Jewelry

Song of Solomon 3:11 KJV Go forth, O ye daughters of Zion, and behold king Solomon with the crown wherewith his mother crowned him in the day of his espousals, and in the day of the gladness of his heart.

Genesis 41:42 NIV Then Pharaoh took his signet ring from his finger and put it on Joseph's finger…and put a gold chain around his neck.

Luke 15:22 NIV But the father said to his servants…put a ring on his finger.

Daniel 5:29 NLT Then at Belshazzar's command, a gold chain was hung around (Daniel's) neck.

Deformities

Let the Loving Father heal you, yes even the smallest thing that is big to you. He loves you. God can heal, restore and make you whole so cast your deformities, at Jesus' feet so you can be made whole. You might not need plastic surgery, you just need God's SUPERNATURAL!

Matthew 15:30-31 KJV [30]And great multitudes came unto him, having with them those that were … maimed (missing body part) … and cast them down at Jesus' feet; and he healed them: [31]Insomuch that the multitude wondered, when they saw … the maimed to be whole (restored body part) and they glorified the God of Israel.

Say this: Jesus I come to you and I lay my (state your deformity) at your feet and I receive my restored body part(s). I give you Glory God in Jesus Name.

Jesus REDEEMED us from The Curse

Galatians 3:13 KJV Christ hath redeemed us from the curse of the law, being made a curse for us: for it is written, Cursed is every one that hangeth on a tree.

Matthew 4:23 KJV (Jesus) healing all kinds of sickness and all kinds of disease.

There is no sickness, diseases or death in Heaven. Thou Kingdom Come Thy Will Be Done on EARTH as it is in Heaven.

God doesn't put sicknesses, diseases, death on people. Satan does!!! Remember Jesus died on the cross, He shed his blood, his body was broken and by His stripes we are healed. Why would he die for us to be healed, healthy, wealthy, get married, have children, have a long life for Him to turn around and bring bad things on us. God is not some Dr. Jekyll and Mr. Hyde. You need to get in the Bible to know who God is which is GOOD!! Research the Bible on all scriptures on the Goodness of God. How can a Good God be Evil?

NOW God is also a JUDGE just like the laws on that earth that needs to be followed there are Kingdom Laws that must be followed with God so if you go against it God will judge just like on earth where if you break laws you may find yourself in front of a judge. That is why it's best to be obedient to God.

PLEASE NOTE you can put sicknesses and diseases on yourself from your own doing by having an unhealthy lifestyle such as what you eat, drink, certain sexual activities (science backs this), unlawful things, unforgiveness (science backs this), fear (science back this), being unrepentant etc. But Jesus! Jesus is so gracious He will heal you so don't feel condemned if you did some things and you got a disease etc. Jesus died on the Cross and He has healing powers in His shed Blood.

Jesus came and sacrificed Himself for us. He shed blood and His body was broken for us to be healed. READ Galatians 3:13 again.

Please see examples of the curse listed from the Bible. You may not see your condition, symptom, pain, disease, sickness listed but you name it in the ACTION STEP to be healed.

The Curse: Skin Condition, Skin Diseases
Deuteronomy 28:27 VOICE The Eternal will afflict you with all kinds of incurable skin diseases, such as the boils that were a plague in Egypt; you'll suffer tumors and scurvy and itch, but you'll never find relief.

The Curse: Hair and Scalp
Isaiah 3:17 NIV sores will be upon your head and balding.

Isaiah 3:24 NLT her elegant hair will fall out.

The Curse: Sickness and Disease
Deuteronomy 28:21-22 NET [21]The Lord will plague you with deadly diseases until he has completely removed you from the land you are about to possess. [22]He will afflict you with weakness, fever, inflammation, infection.

The Curse: No Break at All
Isaiah 3:24 CEV
In place of Perfume, there will be a Stink;
In place of Belts, there will be Ropes;
In place of Fancy Hairdos, they will have Bald Heads.
Instead of Expensive Clothes, they will Wear Sackcloth;
Instead of Beauty, they will have Ugly Scars.

ACTION STEP: Receive Your Healing

For those who have deformities, conditions and/or disease with your **eyesight** and **hearing** receive your healing because according to Proverbs 20:12 ERV It was the LORD who gave us eyes for seeing and ears for hearing.

For all others according to Galatians 3:13 Christ redeemed you from the curse of (Name Your Symptom, Condition, Sickness, Pain, Disease, Deformity) it has to bow in Jesus Name. Restore in Jesus Name creative miracles come. Be healed and be made whole in Jesus Name.

Question for the Day
Does God curse people?

Jun 25, 2019

According to Kenneth Copeland Ministry, "Ephesians 4:27 tells us to not give place to the devil, and disobeying God is one way a Christian can give place to him. Disobedience opens doors to everything from sickness and disease to destruction and death (Romans 6:23). So, one of the keys to keeping Satan and his destruction out of our lives is for us to obey God (1 John 5:18). God is NOT the author of the curse or anything related to the curse, such as sickness, poverty and death (John 10:10). The source of a cursed life is sin, and the source of sin is the devil—not God. Nothing about living a cursed life is willed by God, because His will is clearly revealed through Jesus. Always remember that we serve a good God who looks for ways to bless and not curse us (Psalm 35:27; Proverbs 10:22; Ezekiel 33:11)!" (Question, 83)

Married Couples

Wives

HYGIENE ISSUES

Hygiene can be an issue in Lovemaking especially oral sex maybe you have insecurity about how your vagina smells and especially if you husband mentioned it. Before lovemaking, take a bath or shower.

Song of Solomon 7:8 MSG Your breath is clean and cool like fresh mint

Proverbs 30:12 MSG Don't imagine yourself to be quite presentable when you haven't had a bath in weeks.

Song of Solomon 4:10 NET Bible …the fragrance of your perfume is better than any spice!

SLEEP ISSUES

Sleep is sexy getting rest daily will help your sex life. Your body repairs and heals itself with the proper amount of sleep. Remember wife sex will put you to sleep. Ha!Ha!

Proverbs 3:24 CEV You will rest without a worry and sleep soundly.

Psalm 4:8 NLT In peace I will lie down and sleep, for you alone, O LORD, will keep me safe.

<u>SEX DESIRE ISSUES</u>

You may have a low sex drive, maybe no desire for sex. God has given you Sexual Desires towards your husband. Then wife you take that sexiness and put it on your husband, girl.

Wife to stir up your sexuality
1 Corinthians 7:3 VOICE Each husband has the responsibility to meet his wife's sexual desires, and each wife should do the same for her husband.

1 Corinthians 7:3 AMPC Do not refuse and deprive and defraud each other [of your due marital (sexual) rights] …lest Satan tempt you [to sin] through your lack of restraint of sexual desire.

1 Corinthians 7:34 PHILLIPS The married woman must concern herself with the things of this world, and her aim will be to please her husband.

Initiate Love Making
Proverbs 5:19 TPT Let her breasts be your satisfaction, and let her embrace intoxicate you at all times. Be continually delighted and ravished with her love!

<u>SEXUAL DYSFUNCTION</u>

Lack of Lubrication

Song of Solomon 4:12 KJV A garden inclosed my spouse; a spring shut up, a fountain sealed.

Song of Solomon 4:15 KJV A fountain of gardens, a well of living waters, and streams from Lebanon.

Ask God for your natural sexual lubrication. Continuous sex will help you.

According to Dr. Ja-Hong Kim, "As women get older, their vaginas are prone to losing elasticity and lubrication. This is due to hormonal changes that generally accompany menopause. There is good news, however. "If the woman remains sexually active throughout her life, it [the vagina] retains some of these properties better," says Kim. "It's a use it or lose it kind of thing." Continued stimulation of the vagina can help keep the glands and muscles in working order. The opposite is also true. Kim has seen older women who are not sexually active lose their elasticity to the point that their vaginal opening is restricted to the size of two fingers. (Kubota, 83).

Husbands

<u>HYGIENE ISSUES</u>

Hygiene can be an issue in Lovemaking especially oral sex there maybe some insecurity with sweating down there and maybe your wife complained of your smelly balls. Before lovemaking, take a bath or shower.

Song of Solomon 7:8 MSG Your breath is clean and cool like fresh mint

Proverbs 30:12 MSG Don't imagine yourself to be quite presentable when you haven't had a bath in weeks.

Song of Solomon 1:3 NET The fragrance of your colognes is delightful.

<u>SLEEP ISSUES</u>

Sleep is sexy getting rest daily will help your sex life. Your body repairs and heals itself with the proper amount of sleep. Remember husband sex will put you to sleep. Ha!Ha!

Proverbs 3:24 CEV You will rest without a worry and sleep soundly.

Psalm 4:8 NLT In peace I will lie down and sleep, for you alone, O LORD, will keep me safe.

<u>SEX DESIRE ISSUES</u>

You may have a low sex drive, maybe no desire for sex. God has given you a Yearning for sex toward your wife.

Husband to stir up your sexuality
Psalm 45:11 VOICE Because the king yearns for your beauty

Proverbs 5:19 NLT Let her breasts satisfy you always. May you always be captivated by her love.

Song of Solomon 4:10 DRB How beautiful are thy breasts, my sister, my spouse! thy breasts are more beautiful than wine, and the sweet smell of thy ointments above all aromatical spices.

Vitality / Vigor Even In Old Age
Deuteronomy 34:7 TLB Moses was 120 years old when he died, yet his eyesight was perfect and he was as strong as a young man.

<u>SEXUAL DYSFUNCTION</u>

Impotence
Romans 4:19, 21 MSG [19]Abraham didn't focus on his own impotence and say, "It's hopeless...He didn't tiptoe around God's promise asking cautiously skeptical questions. He plunged into the promise and came up strong, ready for God, [21]sure that God would make good on what he had said.

Psalm 45:3 KJV Gird thy sword upon thy thigh, O most mighty, with thy glory and thy majesty.

Work related stresses to impotence:
Luke 1:23 -24 NASB [23]When the days of his priestly service were concluded, he went back home. [24]Now after these days his wife Elizabeth became pregnant, and she kept herself in seclusion for five months.

Mental Health

God as your Therapist

1 Peter 5:7 NLT Give all your worries and cares to God, for he cares about you.

Seek Counsel

Proverbs 20:18 KJV Every purpose is established by counsel: and with good advice make war.

Proverbs 11:4 KJV Where no counsel is, the people fall: but in the multitude of counsellors there is safety.

Proverbs 12:15 KJV but he that hearkeneth unto counsel is wise.

Proverbs 15:22 KJV Without counsel purposes are disappointed: but in the multitude of counsellors they are established.

Proverbs 19:20 KJV Hear counsel, and receive instruction, that thou mayest be wise in thy latter end.

Proverbs 24:6 KJV For by wise counsel thou shalt make thy war: and in multitude of counsellors there is safety.

Proverbs 1:5 KJV A wise man will hear, and will increase learning; and a man of understanding shall attain unto wise counsels.

Renew your Mind

Philippians 2:5 KJV Let this mind be in you, which was also in Christ Jesus:

1 Corinthians 2:16 KJV For who hath known the mind of the Lord, that he may instruct him? But we have the mind of Christ.

Romans 8:6 KJV For to be carnally minded is death; but to be spiritually minded is life and peace.

Proverbs 23:4 ERV Above all, be careful what you think because your thoughts control your life.

Proverbs 10:7 KJV The memory of the just is blessed.

Philippians 4:8 KJV Finally, brethren, whatsoever things are true, whatsoever things are honest, whatsoever things are just, whatsoever things are pure, whatsoever things are lovely, whatsoever things are of good report; if there be any virtue, and if there be any praise, think on these things.

Break Free from Controlling People

Song of Solomon 1:6 GNT Don't look down on me because of my color, because the sun has tanned me. My brothers were angry with me and made me work in the vineyard. I had no time to care for myself.

1 Corinthians 15:33 NKJV Do not be deceived: "Evil company corrupts good habits."

FOR THE FEMALE "Me Time"

Woman's Nature, Womanhood, Femininity

You need time to connect with other women, spend time with your girlfriends.

Acts 16:13 NIV On the Sabbath we went outside the city gate to the river, where we expected to find a place of prayer. We sat down and began to speak to the women who had gathered there.

FOR THE MALE "Me time"

Man's Nature, Manhood, Warrior nature

You need time to connect with other men, spend time with your boys.

Exodus 15:3 NIV The LORD is a warrior; the LORD is his name.

Etiquette

Proverbs 23:1-3 ERV [1]When you sit and eat with an important person, remember who you are with. [2]Never eat too much, even if you are very hungry. [3]Don't eat too much of his fine food. It might be a trick.

Proverbs 23: 6-7 NLT [6]Don't eat with people who are stingy; don't desire their delicacies. [7]They are always thinking about how much it costs. "Eat and drink," they say, but they don't mean it.

Proverbs 23:20 CEV Don't be a heavy drinker or stuff yourself with food.

Colossians 4:6 NASB Your speech must always be with grace, as though seasoned with salt, so that you will know how you should respond to each person.

1 Corinthians 14:40 KJV Let all things be done decently and in order.

Philippians 4:5 GNT Show a gentle attitude toward everyone.

Galatians 5:22-23 NLT [22]But the Holy Spirit produces this kind of fruit in our lives: love, joy, peace, patience, kindness, goodness, faithfulness, [23]gentleness, and self-control. There is no law against these things!

Proverbs 15:17 GNT Better to eat vegetables with people you love than to eat the finest meat where there is hate.

FEMALE "Manners"

1 Timothy 3:11 GNT states Their wives also must be of good character and must not gossip, they must have self-control and be honest in everything.

MALE "Manners"

1 Timothy 3:2 NIV, 3:3 NLT [2]Now the overseer is to be above reproach, faithful to his wife, temperate, self-controlled, respectable, hospitable, able to teach, [3]He must not be a heavy drinker or be violent. He must be gentle, not quarrelsome, and not love money.

Fitness

Weight Loss
Song of Solomon 7:7 NLT You are slender like a palm tree.

Exercise, Weight Loss
Esther 2:7 CSB The young woman (Esther) had a beautiful figure.

Esther 2:7 NIV This young woman, who was also known as Esther, had a lovely figure.

Exercise
Song of Solomon 2:9 NLT (male) My lover is like a swift gazelle or a young stag.

Song of Solomon 5:10 CSB (male) My love is fit and strong

Mindset
Philippians 4:13 KJV I can do all things through Christ which strengtheneth me.

1 Corinthians 6:19 NLT Don't you realize that your body is the temple of the Holy Spirit, who lives in you and was given to you by God? You do not belong to yourself.

Well-being

Proverbs 17:22 ESV A joyful heart is good medicine, but a crushed spirit dries up the bones.

Exercise

1 Corinthians 9:27 NLT I discipline my body like an athlete, training it to do what it should.

Proverbs 31:17 KJV (female) She girdeth her loins with strength, and strengtheneth her arms.

Dance

Song of Solomon 6:13 CEV Dance! Dance! Beautiful woman from Shulam, let us see you dance! Why do you want to see this woman from Shulam dancing with the others?

Mark 6:22 CEV The daughter of Herodias came in and danced for Herod and his guests.

Healthy Eating

Psalm 103:5 KJV Who satisfieth thy mouth with good things; so that thy youth is renewed like the eagle's.

Philippians 4:5 KJV Let your moderation be known unto all men. The Lord is at hand.

Acts 27:34 KJV Wherefore I pray you to take some meat: for this is for your health.

1 Corinthians 10:31 NIV So whether you eat or drink or whatever you do, do it all for the glory of God.

Esther 2:9 She pleased him and won his favor. Immediately he provided her with her beauty treatments and special food.

Daniel 1:12-13,15 NLT [12]"Please test us for ten days on a diet of vegetables and water," Daniel said. [13]"At the end of the ten days, see how we look compared to the other young men who are eating the king's food… [15]At the end of the ten days, Daniel and his three friends looked healthier and better nourished than the young men who had been eating the food assigned by the king.

Genesis 1:29 NIV Then God said, "I give you every seed-bearing plant on the face of the whole earth and every tree that has fruit with seed in it. They will be yours for food.

John 4:14 NIV But whoever drinks the water I give them will never thirst. Indeed, the water I give them will become in them a spring of water welling up to eternal life.

Ezekiel 4:9 ERV You must get some grain to make bread. Get some wheat, barley, beans, lentils, millet, and spelt. Mix all these things together in one bowl and grind them to make flour. You will use this flour to make bread.

Genesis 43:11 KJV And their father Israel said unto them, If it must be so now, do this; take of the best fruits in the land in your vessels, and carry down the man a present, a little balm, and a little honey, spices, and myrrh, nuts, and almonds.

Lifespan

Live to 120
Then the Lord said, "I will not allow people to live forever; they are mortal. From now on they will live no longer than 120 years. Genesis 6:3 GNT

With long life I will satisfy him and show him my salvation. Psalm 91:16 NIV

Everyone will live a long life. Exodus 23:26 CEV

Restored vision
Moses was one hundred and twenty years old when he died. His eyes were not dim. Deuteronomy 34:7 NKJV

Restored hearing
Ears that hear and eyes that see - we get our basic equipment from God! Proverbs 20:12 MSG

Height Increase
And Jesus increased in... stature. Luke 2:52 KJV

Supernatural Metamorphosis

Body Transformation. God can transform your whole body. Allow God to do supernatural body restoration and renewal from hair, head to toes.

Jesus said, "Anything is possible if a person believes."
Mark 9:23 NLT

2 Corinthians 3:18 NASB But we all, with unveiled faces, looking as in a mirror at the glory of the Lord, are being transformed into the same image from glory to glory, just as from the Lord, the Spirit.

Job 33:25 NLT Then his body will become as healthy as a child's, firm and youthful again.

Job 33:25 GNT Their bodies will grow young and strong again

2 Corinthians 5:17 KJV Therefore if any man be in Christ, he is a new creature: old things are passed away; behold, all things are become new.

Matthew 17:2 HCSB He was transformed in front of them, and His face shone like the sun. Even His clothes became as white as the light.

Exodus 34:29 HCSB It came about when Moses was coming down from Mount Sinai (and the two tablets of the testimony were in Moses' hand as he was coming down from the mountain), that Moses did not know that the skin of his face shone because of his speaking with Him.

Romans 12:2 KJV And be not conformed to this world: but be ye transformed by the renewing of your mind, that ye may prove what is that good, and acceptable, and perfect, will of God.

Luke 24:16,31 TLB [16]But they didn't recognize him, for God kept them from it. [31]when suddenly—it was as though their eyes were opened—they recognized him! And at that moment he disappeared!

Mark 16:12 TLB Later that day he appeared to two who were walking from Jerusalem into the country, but they didn't recognize him at first because he had changed his appearance.

2 Corinthians 5:17 KJV Therefore if any man be in Christ, he is a new creature: old things are passed away; behold, all things are become new.

The Prayer

Allow God to Supernaturally metamorphose your body, healing it and making it whole.

The Bible is about the Supernatural, it's God's nature and the healings were metamorphosis from a broken condition to a restored state which you can receive in your own life now. Blind eyes were open. Closed mouths were open, the mute were able to speak. Age reversal took place where people looked younger to their youth. Skin restored. Hair grew back instantly. People were unrecognizable. People raised from the dead. The maimed are those with deformities that had missing body parts from birth or afterwards which could have come through other means through war, mutilation, disease, sickness, accidents, a person's choice etc. Matthew 4:23 KJV states And Jesus went about all Galilee, teaching in their synagogues, and preaching the gospel of the kingdom, and healing all manner of sickness and all manner of disease among the people.

Allow God to metamorphose your whole body that is Jesus's gift to you. He died on the cross, shed His blood and His body was broken because of that so receive the gift of healing and wholeness.

You may say, "Well Queen Dy I have this big birthmark on my right leg that I hate wearing shorts. I don't want to bother God with that." Jesus loves you and shed His blood for you to be healed so receive it.

You may say, "Well Queen Dy I was born with this condition, symptom, disease, impediment, it's in my family DNA." Jesus died on the cross shed His blood for you to be healed. He is releasing His DNA in you to restore what you got from your family bloodline. It could be a generational curse that filtering through your bloodline for example heart disease started with your great-great grandfather and the possibility or probability are that you will have it but Jesus's blood can heal that.

You may say, "Hey Dy I thought this healing stuff was only in the Bible." No, because God healed me of thyroid problem, the right was taken out and I would have taken pills the rest of my life but I don't have to do that. I had an enlarged heart. I had to get cardiac catheterization and they put me on high blood pressure pills and even a statin. God healed me and I don't take either. I had gotten an x-ray and it revealed my heart was enlarged but years later for another x-ray for a totally different reason my doctor gave me the vitals and out of know where she said your heart is not enlarged. This was a different doctor from years ago when it was diagnosed. I was praising God for healing me. Some of these were simultaneously in my life and at separate seasons in my life but God healed me. So many stories of Jesus healing I even gave Glory to God in a book I wrote many years ago about Him healing me of other ailments, sicknesses and disease and yes even some of the same one He had healed me of previously. Yes some of it was my ignorance "My Fault" but the others it could have been because of family line DNA, environmental conditions, just plain ole satan sending infirmity spirits attacking my body and witchcraft too. Jesus healing is there right now He is a present help in your time of need.

"Dy, I know you are not saying God can restore my hair, I read in the book where you showed He did it for Samson but for me, no way." Yes God can do it. I had short hair and God grew it. I had a real ponytail, "Black Girl Ponytail" and it was my hair, my real hair then with the thyroid issue my hair broke off and it was brittle. Funny but not funny it started breaking off on the right side where I had the thyroid problem so I don't know if that has any significance. Then it grew back. I started going to a professional instead of doing my own hair and she showed me the excessive curling ironing was damaging my hair. I even wouldn't go back when she suggested so the hair would grow and the old growth would pop off at the line of demarcation because the hair did not get moisture. I got new growth but the old popped off. At that time I was using a relaxer. I got educated because I wasn't taking care of my hair. I had to resort to weaves but I just later went to wigs. As you can see God was blessing me but I was destroying my own blessing. My people are destroyed for lack of knowledge (Hosea 4:6). Then there are incidents God revealed to me witchcraft was done against my hair.

"Dy, I am not a Christian." Who do you think Jesus healed when He was on earth? No one became Believers until after He went to Heaven. Girl! Boy! Get your healing. No Excuse.

Reader, you know what you want; it may seem outlandish to others but not to God. Jesus said if you can believe then all things are possible to those who believe Mark 9:23.

Now let me release the prayer over you so you can receive what God promised you, a new healed, whole, body where nothing is missing and nothing is broken, a Hebrew term "Shalom" in Jesus Name.

Abba Father in the name of Jesus I command your hand according to Isaiah 45:11 to stretch forth according to Acts 4:30 upon the reader's body to metamorphose it. Thou Kingdom Come thy will be done from the top of their heads down to the soles of their feet.

Matthew 15:30-31 KJV [30]And great multitudes came unto him, having with them those that were lame, blind , dumb, **maimed {missing body parts}**, and many others, and cast them down at Jesus' feet; and he healed them: [31]Insomuch that the multitude wondered, when they saw the dumb to speak, **the maimed to be whole {restored body part}**, the lame to walk, and the blind to see: and they glorified the God of Israel.

Abba Father, stretch forth Your hand upon every deformities Matthew 15:31 KJV people came for healing who were maimed which mean missing body parts and Jesus healed them and the missing body parts were restored and instantly they received new limbs miraculously supernatural. Perform creative miracles on the reader's body metamorphosing their body whole in Jesus Name.

Abba Father stretch forth your hand on their HAIR & SCALP going deep in the epidermis, dermis and subcutaneous fat levels rejuvenating the blood supply to nutrify the hair, strengthening the hair strands, preventing inflammation, awakening the dead hair follicles, opening closed hair follicles, reappearing disappeared hair follicles, restoring damaged and scarred hair follicles, restoring the two hair follicles, regenerating new hair follicles. Restore the short, thin, weak, brittle, dry, damaged, coarse, wiry and dull hair, hair breakage and loss, baldness, all forms of scalp diseases and conditions such as psoriasis, dandruff, candida etc. Restore the hair and scalp to a healthy condition. Allow the hair to grow instantly just like Samson, Judges 16:22 KJV Howbeit the hair of his head began to grow again. Recall all lost hairs they are out there in molecules Luke 12:7 even the very hairs of my head are all numbered. Perform creative miracles for those who want long hair, full hair, thick hair, soft hair, silky hair, sheeny hair, shiny hair, moisturized hair and scalp, hydrated hair and scalp, knot free hair and split-end free hair. 1 Corinthians 11:15 NKJV but if a woman has long hair, it is a glory to her; for her hair is given to her for a covering. 2 Samuel 14:26 GNT His hair was very thick, and he had to cut it once a year, when it grew too long and heavy. It would weigh about five pounds according to the royal standard of weights.

Abba Father stretch forth your hand on their FACE & BODY going deep in their SKIN in the epidermis, dermis, hypodermis levels removing Dermatosis Papulosa Nigra, Seborrheic Keratoses, Acanthosis Nigricans, Dermatofibromas, Moles, Scars, Pimples, Freckles, Keloids, Skin Pigmentation Disorders, Inflammation, Uneven Toned Skin, Stretchmarks, Cellulite, Vitiligo, Centrofacial Neurodysraphic Lentiginosis, Leopard skin, Noonan Syndrome, Liver Spots, Skin Tags, Dark Pubic Area, Velvet Skin, Sun Damage, any and all skin conditions and skin diseases according to Mark 11:23. Restore their skin to their youth eventoned, blemish free, flawless and clear. Job 33:25 let their flesh be renewed like a child let them be restored as the days of their youth. 2 Kings 5:14 and his flesh were restored like the flesh of a little child and he was clean. 2 Samuel 14:25 from the top of his head to the soles of his feet there was no blemish in him. Psalm 103:5 your youth is restored like the Eagles. Song of Solomon 7:2 MSG our skin is like silk.

Abba Father stretch forth Your hand on their mouth creative miracle on their teeth for a full set of healthy, white straight teeth. Missing teeth restored. Cavities and Filling be gone, creative miracle restored teeth. Song of Solomon 4:2 CEV Your teeth are whiter than sheep freshly washed; they match perfectly, not one is missing. Crooked teeth, straighten! Restore their breath from halitosis and dry mouth Song of Solomon 7:8 MSG Your breath is clean and cool like fresh mint.

Abba Father stretch forth Your hand upon their body creative miracles for the overweight person, shrink their body fat to the perfect weight for their height and frame. Creative miracles removing all sagging skin giving them tight and toned skin. For the underweight person increase their weight to the perfect size for their height and frame.

- New body parts, Come! Reader, call out that body part you are believing for.
- Hot Flashes, Go!
- Cosmetics scar, Go!
- Scar tissue, Restore!
- Sagging skin, Tighten!
- Uncontrollable Sweating, Stop!
- Missing teeth, Come!
- Crooked teeth, Straighten!
- Wrinkles, Go!
- Sun damaged skin, Go!
- Turkey neck, Tighten!
- Jawline, Tone!
- Yellow, Brown Gray teeth, Whiten!
- Eyelids, Lift! God's cosmetic surgery.
- Booty, Lift!
- Boobs, lift, perky breasts, Come!
- Dark circle under eyes, Lighten!
- Receding Hairline, Restore!
- Gravity reversed! Sagging and drooping, Be Thou Removed!
- Liver, gallbladder, and pancreas, RESTORE!!
- Feet, Restore!
- Microbiome, Restore!
- Genitals, Restore! from Sexual Abuse! Be Healed and Be Made Whole!!!

Abba Father stretch forth Your hand release your vengeance, judgment on every demon, devils and all its ranks (Ephesians 6:12) and witches (the occultists) sending attacks, infirmities spirits, torment, demonic prayers, declaration, using witchcraft altars and covens all attacking the reader's body internally and externally. Bind all attacks and return it back to the sender. Restore the reader's body in Jesus Name.

Reader, if I didn't state your condition in the book, use your faith to call out the sicknesses, diseases, missing body parts, pain, trauma, impediment you want healed, restored and made whole now as you are reading this. Remember: Jesus <u>healing all manner of sickness and all manner of disease</u> among the people. Then say, "I receive it!"

Write down what you are believing God for:

____

____

____

____

Reader, now I want you to do the impossible, move that body part that you were having issues with. If you have a limp walk, if you have pain check it, if you have a growth or rash check it. If you couldn't jump, jump. Do what you couldn't do. If you have an addiction, notice that desire is gone. Take an Act of Faith by walking, moving, and checking to see.

Thank God for your healing and deliverance.

Then share your testimony how God did it. Take the after pictures, use them as "Show and Tell" to tell the goodness of God to others. Freely you receive Freely you give Matthew 10:8. Sometimes just sharing your story releases faith in others and even they are being healed as well.

WARNING:

Don't stop your medicines until you get checked by your doctor to get the documented proof.

Reference

"Question of the Day: Does God curse people?" Kenneth Copeland Ministries, 25 June 2019, www.kcm.org/read/question-of-the-day/does-god-curse-people. Accessed 13 September 2022.

Kubota, Taylor. "12 Things Everyone Should Know About Vaginas." Men's Journal, www.mensjournal.com/health-fitness/12-things-everyone-should-know-about-vaginas-20150114. Accessed 13 September 2022.

In Closing...

Immerse yourself in the word and receive your body's total metamorphosis from God.

You are precious to God, Jesus and the Holy Ghost so receive all He has.

Be Blessed!!

Give

The one who is taught the word [of God] is to share all good things with his teacher [contributing to his spiritual and material support]. Galatians 6:6 AMP

If you were blessed by the teaching in this book Galatians 6:6 states that you can give to the teacher.

Please pray to God if He would like for you to give and if He says yes then ask Him how much you should give.

If you are giving, please wrap your faith with your giving. Your faith is what you have been meditating on, scriptures, from this book. **As you give, say "I receive."** Make notation of your giving.

I speak over your giving. "May God bless you with a hundredfold in Jesus Name." I thank you for the gift, I receive it and God Bless You.

Ways to Give:
https://www.globalbusinessqueens.com/give.html

https://www.paypal.com/paypalme/DyWakefield

https://www.paypal.com/donate/?hosted_button_id=W5SSEDEHUM26G

Contact

Website: www.DyWakefield.com
Website: www.GlobalBusinessQueens.com

Social Media
Facebook: www.facebook.com/DyWakefield
Twitter: www.twitter.com/DyWakefield
Instagram: www.instagram.com/DyWakefield
YouTube: www.youtube.com/@dywakefield
YouTube: www.youtube.com/@dythequeen

Send Testimonies to email:
whereveryousetfoot@yahoo.com

Miracle Healing and Deliverance Prayer

Abba Father in Jesus Name I call you as Jehovah Rapha the God who heals and as Jehovah Mephalti the God who delivers. I command your hand to stretch forth upon this reader. Father, release your healing, miracles, signs, wonders, and deliverance angels. Holy Spirit, fall right now wherever the reader is and heal and cure them.

Reader, the anointing of God will come upon your head to your feet and saturate your body, heal you and minister to you. The anointing will go in your body and destroy the yoke of bondage making the infirmities, sicknesses, diseases, pain, addictions leave. Lay hand on that part of the body and call out the issue its name because it has to bow in Jesus Name.

I demand every cell, bones, organs and tissues in your body to line up with the Word of God. I bind every demon and cast them out to the lake of fire. Some will leave because of the anointing but the others won't because you are giving them permission to stay.

Reader, you need to renounce those demons inside of you to be set free, don't keep some and get rid of the rest. Totally surrender to the anointing and let them all go by saying, "I renounce all demons and blood covenants. I sever ties from them and the people I am wrongly involved with."

I bind the spirits of Jannes and Jambres. I bind messengers of satan, seducing spirits, doctrines of devils and infirmity spirits. I bind all and any forms of witchcraft, clairvoyance, and astral projecting that was done to you. I bind all and any forms of witchcraft off this reader and their family.

Reader, right now call out a family member, loved one, spouse, child, friend etc.

Abba Father release your vengeance and return every curse sent upon the reader back to sender 100-fold. I call fire from Heaven upon satanic altars with the reader's pictures, names, addresses, DNA samples, clothing, effigies, voodoo dolls of their image. Let the blood of Jesus nullify that. I bind and break curses sent with words "over my dead body" and return it back to the sender. I bind and cancel all demonic dreams such as recruiting, monitoring, mind controlling, mind reading, evil eye, entering in demonic partnerships, contracts, marriages, blood covenant, creating demonic spiritual babies and children with demons, sexual activity, perverse activities, paralysis. I bind and cancel demonically infiltrating music, miscarriages, sterileness, birth defects, premature deaths, fears, sicknesses and diseases through dreams. I bind demonically administering drinks, food, foreign substances, drugs, etc. in dreams.

Jesus, transcend back to the reader as a baby in the womb and heal the soul wounds.

I bind all demons and I loose them back to the sender bringing great fear, great dread, great tremble and great torment upon the sender and then I cast the demons to the lake of fire. I decree the wealth of the wicked "the sender" will come to the reader in Jesus Name.

Be healed, be made whole, **RESTORE** in Jesus Name. New body parts come! Creative Miracles come!

Reader, now I want you to do the impossible, move that body part that you were having issues with. If you have a limp walk, if you have pain check it, if you have a growth or rash check it. If you couldn't jump, jump. Do what you couldn't do. If you have an addiction, notice that desire is gone. Take an Act of Faith by walking, moving, and checking to see.

Deliverance:
There's another step to deliverance and it's about you repenting of your sins and forgiving those who hurt you. Holy Spirit, reveal the sins they need to confess so they can be cleansed of it.

Holy Ghost, reveal to them those they need to forgive. Reader, it may be hard to forgive so you have to ask Jesus to give you that spirit to forgive. You are <u>only</u> forgiving those people through confession to God, you are not going to them and saying I forgive you, you heathen. Your forgiveness is a release from that hurt, a form of bondage holding you trapped in your life. Receive the Times of Refreshing from the Lord Acts:3:20.

Start here in your confessions:
- Abba Father, I repent of (state the sins) I receive my forgiveness and cleansing in Jesus Name.
- Abba Father, I forgive (state their names). I bless them and I release them to you in Jesus Name.

Abba Father I soak this reader's soul with the Power of the Cross, the Power of the Resurrection, the Blood of Jesus, the Dunamis Power, the Glory Light of Jesus, the Holy Ghost Fire, the Fire of God and Thundering of God in their soul producing Excellence of Soul. Whom the Son makes free is free indeed John 8:36. God cut them free from the cord of wickedness Psalm 129:4.

PLEASE NOTE: Healing can come instantly or gradually. Your part is to thank God for your healing.

WARNING: Don't stop your medicines until you get checked by your doctor to get the documented proof.

Salvation

If you're tired of trying to do things your way in life, how about giving Jesus a try? Ask Jesus to be the Lord and Savior over your life surrendering all to Him. Allow Him to come into your heart. Be sincere. Be fed up with how your life is going now and tell Jesus you are ready to receive Him, His love, protection, help, deliverance and healing. All I ask is for you to just try Him, your life will never be the same.

Say this, "Jesus, come into my heart, I am tired of living the life I am living now. I confess that you died on the cross for my sins and rose again by the Holy Spirit. Jesus, I choose you to be the Lord and Savior over my life."

To the Believer who finds yourself far from the truth I bind deception and I loose clarity. Don't feel condemned, Jesus still loves you. He died for you. Come back into the Father's loving arms. Please repent so your sins will be blotted out so that the "Times of Refreshing" will come.

I just want to acknowledge that God sent Jesus the Messiah the Chosen One for you. When you confess your sins to God, your sins are washed away by the blood of Jesus. He is no longer angry with you if you accept this Gospel message.

Baptized in the Holy Spirit

PLEASE NOTE: You must be saved or in other words you must have accepted Jesus Christ as your Lord and Savior by confessing that with your mouth before you can be baptized in the Holy Spirit.

ACTION STEP

If you like to be Baptized in the Holy Spirit with the ability of speaking in tongues Say this: "Holy Ghost I desire that gift of Speaking in Tongues and I receive it thank you."

The Holy Ghost will guide you in this beautiful language that will bring you intimately to God.

Holy Ghost loose this reader's tongue.

God as Your Business Partner

Your business is not where you want it to be, how about giving Jesus a try? Do you know there are many business people in the Bible? In the Old Testament there is Abraham, Issaac, Jacob, Job, Boaz all had business in agriculture plus many others including women. In the New Testament the disciples Peter, James, John and Andrews were all fishermen, Matthew a tax collector, Apostle Paul a tentmaker plus many others including women.

Make a decision today to allow God to take over and help you increase abundantly so you can enjoy the fruits of it with your family. Allow Him to lead you to prosper (teach you to profit Isaiah 48:17).

Say this: "Jesus, I choose you to be the Lord over my businesses so God I am asking that You, Jesus and the Holy Ghost be my Business Partners."

Repent for Wrong Business Practices

NOW Queen if you have been doing wrong business practices in your businesses it's time to get right. Get right with God. Abba Father, remove the scales from this Queen's eyes so she can see and know truth.

Queen, pray this prayer:
"Father, I repent for doing and allowing wrong business practices in my businesses I stop today. I take full responsibility for my actions and my employees. I receive my forgiveness and cleansing. Father, you are all knowing and omniscient so I ask you to be my business partner. I will be led by your spirit, the Holy Spirit as You download ideas, concepts, solutions, and witty inventions through Him to me. I will give you glory in all I do in Jesus Name. I forgive myself and I receive your love. I will be led by the Holy Ghost to remove the dishonest practices from my businesses in Jesus Name."

Queen don't trip, we all make mistakes we all have lived for that DOLLAR you are on the right track now.

You no longer have to work hard for that DOLLAR watch God show you how to multiply to create millions with ease and have balance in your life.

Show Your Commitment

Think about committing to giving financially to God trusting Him with your Business by honoring Him back because what you commit to God He will bless. You just pray to God about that and let Him direct you in your giving. Luke 6:38 TLB For if you give, you will get! Your gift will return to you in full and overflowing measure, pressed down, shaken together to make room for more, and running over. Whatever measure you use to give—large or small—will be used to measure what is given back to you."

As a Business Partner God can direct you in the right products and services, right pricing levels for your products and services, who to hire and who not to hire, who to fire, who to have as clients or who not to deal with. God can reveal things to you that you cannot discern with your eyes. Let God lead you and watch Him accelerate your business.

One thing to remember, do not forget that God is the one that gave you this wisdom and enablement. Praise God in all you do. Always share your testimony to others of the Goodness of God in your life.

Global Business Queens Support

https://www.globalbusinessqueens.com/support.html

I am asking for **supporters** on a continuous basis to support my **Global Vision** to Empower Women in Business. There will be projects, events, traveling and so much more in the making. Be inspired by the free teaching materials on the website and the social medias that it may bring success in your life.

Dy's vision:
Empower, Train and Create over a Million Wealthy Business
Queens Impacting Communities Globally.

Each month I will email you a Business & Empowerment MP3 and monthly letter to empower you in your business or start-up and for personal encouragement. Also, via email I will let you know what projects, events and traveling I am doing and its updates. **You will be informed of what we've done, what we are doing and what we're going to do.** You will always be in my DAILY prayers. **Thank you, you're beautiful!** I will not take this investment lightly because you work hard for it.

About the Author Dy

Dy Wakefield, The Queen of Wealth Advice™ is an Advisor, Multi-Genre Author, Multi-Social Entrepreneur, Speaker, and Aviation Enthusiast.

BUSINESS CREDENTIALS

In 2020 God inspired Dy to transition to Advisor so she took her seat on her Royal Throne.

She was the founder of the now defunct companies Wealthy Woman Dy Investments, Inc., Dy Wakefield International, LLC., Empowering You Events, LLC. Two Biblically Sexually Explicit companies Pleasure Your Husband and Pleasure Your Wife. She was also 51% share partner in Oglesby Concrete Specialists, LLC. Finally, an independent Multi-Level Marketer in Youngevity, a Health MLM, she wanted to bring a sense of Health incorporating a balance of Wealth and Health in her domain.

She has written over 100 books and you can check out her Amazon Author Page where she was blessed to use Amazon publishing as a tool to help her become an author and be creative experimenting in many different genres.

Dy also had four radio shows: The Wealthy Woman Dy Morning Show, Pleasure Your Husband Radio, Pleasure Your Wife Radio and Comfort & Hope in the Midst Radio.

Dy has over 20 years in Accounting, Bookkeeping, Tax Preparations, Business Start-Up and Notary Services. Dy received her BS in Accounting from Clemson University and a Master in Finance specializing in Financial Planning from Kaplan University now Purdue University Global.

Queen Dy's passion for helping women stemmed from personal experience of being underpaid and underappreciated in Corporate America. She wants to break the cycle by helping birth out leaders. 'Dy' is the acronym for "delivery" and she calls herself the midwife for business women. Being a double minority Black and Woman, Dy at times felt like she was at the bottom of the totem pole but she knows that it is God's grace and faith that elevate you not what society has limited you.

PURPOSE/MISSION

Dy has dedicated her life to Empower Women by **Awakening the Queen inside** to be Leaders to own businesses and to be world changers. To help them achieve their destiny through a balanced life and excellence.

Dy has dedicated her life to Empower Wives by **Awakening the Sexual Prowess inside** for their husbands, 1 Corinthians 7:3 NLT version states the husband should Fulfill his Wife's Sexual Needs. God has given Wives' Sexual Needs. There is an inner Sex Vixen that you haven't tapped into. It's your feminine nature to be turned on. Sex & Sex Drive is a Gift from God so "Sex is not dirty it's Pleasurable." Sex is to be enjoyed by both satisfying each other's needs. Ooo La La! You came into a covenant with God and your husband so it's not an emotional thing but a mutual agreement to shake them sheets on a continual basis.

This is a sisterhood to **EMPOWER. TRAIN. CREATE** to be Wealthy and Healthy. A focus on the importance of balance in **FAITH, FAMILY, FITNESS, FINANCE and FUN** as women embrace the role of Queen ruling and reigning in their business Queendom.